Hollywood Beautiful: The Ultimate Hollywood Beauty Secrets and Tips Guide

by Neo Monefa

CLICK THIS LINK TO CLAIM YOUR 100% FREE GIFT !

Table of Contents

1. Introduction
2. Top Celebrity Beauty Secrets
3. Natural Face Masks
4. Anti-Cellulite Tips
5. Anti-Aging Solutions
6. Hollywood Hair Care
7. Detox Weight Loss Programs
8. Top Celebrity Diet Secrets
9. Conclusion

1. Introduction

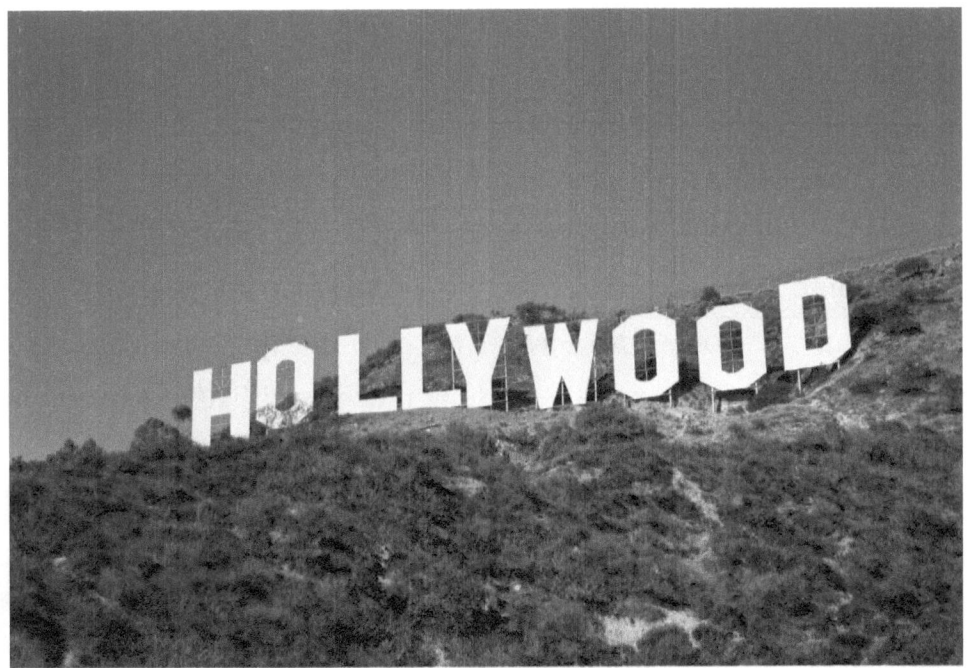

For some of us Hollywood is just an almost surreal far-away land that we can only catch a glimpse of through movies, videos, and advertisements. However we sometimes forget that celebrities whom we may be romancing excessively are normal real people with flesh and blood. We are used to admiring many Hollywood celebrities and maybe some of us even compare ourselves to them. How many times have you been convinced that you are more beautiful or in better shape than a Hollywood celeb? How many times have you thought their hair or skin looks much better than yours? Of course sometimes it may come down to 'make-up tricks' ...however it would be unfair and a bit ridiculous to say that all beauty that can be found in Hollywood is only artificial. Quite often that beauty we admire is not completely a 'natural' endowment, either. Which is the truth then?

The answer is multifaceted and it's definitely something you should know. Why? Because you don't really want to risk falling into feelings of envy or sadness when seeing Hollywood stars shine. People sometimes find it hard to experience pure admiration when they see something they would like to have. So what is the solution to your constant impression that Hollywood beauty is only a distant ideal? You should trust the fact that no celebrity has 100% perfect skin or eye-catching hair as such. Few personalities are actually fit without making any effort. Once you realize Hollywood beauty is often 'shaped' by human hands via intelligent and creative tips, you can stop seeing it as something impossible to reach by a 'common person'. Hollywood beauty is often carefully crafted and mastered, but the means are not only plastic surgery, as you may think.

This book will show you what beauty tips various celebrities use. It will introduce you to concrete methods of improving skin, hair, and weight. After reading this book, you will know what effective natural beauty tips Hollywood celebrities use and you will be able to take direct action in order to improve your own looks. The benefits of having a whole series of already tried and tested beauty tips at your disposal in one single book are undeniable and self-understood. You can trust that the methods used by well-known celebrities are reliable and unique, since hardly any star would have any interest to present to the public tips whose effectiveness is debatable. Considerably more than a 'normal' individual, a famous personality has quite often the advantage of getting advice from many great specialists in natural beauty. What for common people would be much too expensive to get is usually accessible to Hollywood celebrities. Moreover, a famous personality who is admired for their beauty has a form of 'responsibility' in front of the public: a star has a higher standard to meet when presenting working beauty solutions. Why? Because a celebrity can't really afford coming up with a mediocre or banal idea. Given the often drastic competition that reins in Hollywood, when making their beauty tips public and discussing how they maintain their aura and charm, celebrities often have to prove their solutions are at least as good as others'. For all these reasons many beauty tips from Hollywood personalities are particularly reliable.

This book is a guide to the improvement of your beauty according to Hollywood experts. Obviously you shouldn't want to look exactly like a specific celebrity, for self-love is also extremely important. However you can absolutely improve the beauty you already have by using organic solutions. High quality is guaranteed because they are adopted and recommended by renowned personalities whose looks are also quite amazing more often than not. What this book offers you is not only a solution to your need for improvement, but also a unique and valuable approach centered on organic remedies and products. Moreover, in order to meet your complex needs, this beauty guide includes various skin care and hair care ideas as well as a few suggestions for weight loss that Hollywood celebrities have experimented with and found remarkable. Many stars love talking about diets that helped them reach the body shape they have and sharing their effective solutions is as a matter of pride for them.

Without a doubt you will find a myriad of useful tips in this book. It is essential that you read all of these recommendations and decide which of them works the best for your particular needs. Do you currently have weight problems? Are you looking for anti-aging ideas? All you have to do is go through this book and try out the various tips and tactics. Of course you don't have to put everything in practice at once ...but don't hesitate to address what is problematic in your life right now. Instead of wasting your time searching online for random tips whose source in unreliable, now you can find plenty of useful advice in one single book. Start with immediate issues and gradually put the rest in practice, too.

You will see the results on your own and you will save not only time, but also money. As you can imagine, celebrities are rich enough to afford almost anything. How could their beauty tips not be top notch and high quality when most likely they were recommended by specialists? Don't limit yourself to admiring Hollywood celebrities from a distance. Read this book and start using the tips you will find in its pages today.

2. Top Celebrity Beauty Secrets

It is of course important to keep up with fashion and cosmetic trends in Hollywood by means of modern products and clothing style. If Hollywood beauty is your ideal standard, you shouldn't ignore any tips that are communicated directly by celebrities. Keep in mind feeding and treating the fundamental level of beauty (namely the skin) via organic solutions is just as vital. You cannot just cover up your skin with the most up-to-date foundation suggested by Hollywood celebrities if your skin is not actually healthy and radiant. Many celebrities have to use sophisticated make-up most of the time – significantly more than a normal person. For this reason they can hardly afford neglecting the needs of their skin and they choose the best products for deep skin care. You can certainly be sure their organic beauty tips are carefully thought out and quality, since they couldn't afford using mediocre cream or not nourishing their skin properly.

For instance, **Eminence** is the favorite skin care line of many Hollywood stars. Megan Fox whose skin is remarkable confessed the sweet red rose skin cleanser produced by this skin care line is part of her daily routine. Eminence relies only on naturally organic ingredients. Its healing and nourishing effects are high, given its powerful vitamin content as well.

Jennifer Anniston, Nicole Kidman, and Jennifer Lopez intensively use a special cream that makes their skin bright and healthy.

John Masters Organics is a top cosmetic line for Hollywood taste. You may be surprised, but these are high-end products for a reasonable price, so you don't have to worry about breaking the bank in order to be able to afford such skin care. The splendid Zooey Dechanel said she uses the Pomegranate Facial Nourishing Oil produced by this extraordinary line. This oil improves skin elasticity and it draws on 12 organic plants and essential oils. It is great for massage, since it hydrates and nourishes the skin to the fullest. It can be used for the whole body, not just for facial care. Jessica Alba is a huge fan of the Morrocan Clay Purifying mask produced by the same cosmetic line. It has anti-inflammatory properties and it also regulates the balance of oil in the skin without drying it. It is based on pure clay and it uses organic sunflower oil to prevent moisture loss.

Another top line that makes up Hollywood secrets is **Dr. Hauschka**. Many celebrities have mentioned it briefly when asked what they owe their marvelous skin to. Some of them offered details that you are welcome to use to your own advantage. For example, Jennifer Anniston's preferred product is called Radiant You, a special cream produced by Dr.

Hauschka Skin Care. This whole beauty line uses high-quality minerals and plants and it has a very potent natural nourishing effect. Its special cream replenishes delicate layers of the skin and perfectly balances its oil content, while softening and soothing the skin at the same time. Jennifer Lopez and Nicole Kidman recommend the Rose Day Cream, a rich and intensive moisturizer for dry skin. This cream contains no synthetic ingredients. Its formula is designed to soothe irritated or damaged skin. It is a luxurious product that polishes the skin with carefully chosen nutrients. Anne Hathaway who is not only breathtaking through her unique facial features, but also through the doubtless quality and beauty of her skin, she is also among the open fans of this cosmetic line. She confessed she uses multiple products to take care of her skin: the cleanser, the toner, and the moisturizer produced by Dr. Hauschka to make up her daily skin care. When her skin looks so amazing, how could you not trust her tips?

A worldwide appreciated cosmetic line based on thermal water is **Avene**. For instance, Avene is what works best for a contemporary artist like Rita Ora who is in full spotlight. She uses the Avene Thermal Water Spray to hydrate and refresh her skin. The famous Avene thermal water is deeply soothing for all kinds of skin, but you should use it especially if you have problematic or sensitive skin.

Olay is in the kit of many celebrities, from Brittany Snow to Sienna Gomez. The Oil of Olay face and wash lotion is what Sienna Gomez uses to keep her skin healthy, although she knows it is conceived as a product meant to combat aging. She thinks it's so good that it should be used even in youth for its amazing benefits. Brittany Snow uses a wide variety of products in this cosmetic line and she is extremely satisfied with their efficiency on skin. She could hardly find something as good for both dry and oily areas. This product was recommended by her dermatologist and she confirms its quality

An appreciated product for the whole body, Skin Food by **Weleda** is among the favorite beauty products used by Rihanna, Adele, and Victoria Beckham. It is created to moisturize and hydrate dry or rough skin. Its secret is a high quantity of vitamin E and essential fatty acids as well as organic rosemary and calendula extracts which reduce skin inflammation and are known for their anti-septic properties. Reese Witherspoon mentioned that **Vita C Max One Minute Facial** is among her top beauty secrets. Personally she prefers cream rich in vitamin C and this may be the main reason why her skin looks so young and glowing. The product she recommended to the public is extremely special because it draws on seven different types of vitamin C. Its properties are complex: not only does it cleanse your skin, but also it moisturizes and tones it. A definitely intriguing product!

Juice Beauty Green Apple Moisturizer is a preference shared by many Hollywood celebrities and for very good reason. It combines sun protection with organic fruit antioxidants, and coenzyme Q10. It is a light day moisturizer which also reduces fine lines. You can now understand why it is loved so much by stars such as Madonna, Cameron Diaz, or Kate Hudson. A magical product, the **100% Pure Argan Oil by Rosy Maran** is praised by many celebrities who have tried it and use it consistently. It is lightweight and at the same time very rich in vitamin E which nourishes the skin in-depth and gives it a vivid glow. Alicia Silverstone and Julianne Moore are among its most ardent admirers. This product looks like a bona fide skin care health potion. Its producer is an actress herself who knows quite well how high the demands of the glamorous, but very health-oriented Hollywood life are and how much competition her beauty line has to face. Some of the world's best anti-aging solutions, **Intraceuticals**, is wholeheartedly recommended by Victoria Beckham. She uses products for skin brightening and rejuvenation e.g. Rejuvenate Booster serums. They are great for making the skin clearer and lighter and they are also a notable plumping tip.

Gwyneth Paltrow only apparently has perfect skin without doing anything to improve her own looks. It is probably part of her innocent Lolitesque appearance that may make you think she's got eternally young-looking and naturally perfect skin. Remember: Hollywood doesn't give anyone immortality of absolute beauty. What it does offer most celebrities is the drive to be even more beautiful and to avoid letting their lifestyle affect their skin. That's why when you see how pure and beautiful the skin of someone like Paltrow looks, you shouldn't ask yourself how come some people were born perfect. Instead you should gather as much info as you can about their skin care routines. Gwyneth Paltrow said she is captivated by the quality of **Miracle Skin Transformer**, her personal beauty secret. She uses this line for imperfection blurring and skin tinting. She also praised the hydrating and UV protective properties of this product; it contains a large amount of antioxidants that nourish the skin deeply. Raquel Castaneda, a celebrity make-up artist who knows many secrets hidden behind Hollywood beauty recommends drinking plenty of water to ensure skin hydration and using a rich moisturizing cream as well. Her tip is the **Embrioles All—in-One Moisturizer** which in her opinion can meet the demands of many types of skin.

Jessica Alba recommends the luxury line **Vapour** which includes not only skin care products, but also make-up. Gisele

Bundchen shared her own secret: **RMS beauty**. She insisted on her preference for natural brands and confessed she rarely uses chemically-laden products. Alicia Silverstone informed the public that she is very fond of **Tami Fender epi peel** (her scrub tip) and **Crazy Rumors Hibiscus Tinted Lip Balms** which are rich in organic jojoba oil, shea butter and olive oil. Natalie Portman is a fan of the **Ahava Dead Sea Mud Exfoliator** and she also uses the intensive hydration mask produced by the same line. Her solution for keeping her skin bright and healthy is Arcona booster serum. Kate Hudson shared her shower and bathing routines that make her skin look healthier and feel smoother. She prefers using **Elemis Pro Collagen Marine Cream, By Terry Balm, Dr. Bronner Castille Lavander Soap, and Epicurean Coconut Afterbath Moisturizer**. All these products are not only the actress' perfect beauty secret, but also they envelop the body and spirit in a unique atmosphere that delights the senses.

Some celebrities have created their own beauty lines out of a love for organic beauty products. Such an example is Miranda Kerr who invested in Kora Organics, a line that makes use of natural nourishing substances extracted from noni fruit and rosehip seed. Gisele Bundchen launched her own line, Sejaa Skincare. It includes products made of ginseng, green tea, argan oil, and aloe vera natural extracts (day moisturizer, night cream, and clay mask).

3. Natural Face Masks

Although you may think Hollywood figures are so rich, that they can afford buying anything, including the best skin care products on the international market, you should know that quite many celebrities still use natural masks, too. Their choice is obviously based on the rare nourishing quality of such solutions that complement cream, tonic water, or other 'ready-made' products they purchase from certain cosmetic lines.

For instance, Emma Watson uses a mixture of papaya and honey (half cup and one teaspoon, respectively) for her skin care. Anne Hathaway prefers the more 'simple' mask that combines one banana with honey (2 tablespoons). Rachel Bilson confessed her skin has very low tolerance for chemically-laden products and for this reason she prefers treating her skin with something purely organic, namely organic virgin coconut oil whose fatty acids can also be found in the human skin, so its action is one of feeding the skin with its own lost natural oils. She found this solution for keeping your skin soft and preventing water loss much better than a series of famous products. The famous beauty Aishwarya Rai didn't hesitate to admit that she mostly uses natural masks to keep her skin healthy. Her secret weapons are cucumber, milk, and yoghurt to cleanse and moisturize her skin. Her tip for removing toxins is a lotion made up of honey, hot water, and lemon that she uses every morning.

Hayden Panettiere uses a mixture of clove lemon, water, and vinegar to wash her face, since this is an easy solution for acne-affected skin. Beyonce recommends strawberries applied directly on the face as often as possible, especially if you have oily skin. Kim Kardashian's exfoliating tip comes down to nothing more than a spoonful of sugar. She said it is what makes her skin glow and she also uses it for the whole body, not only for facial skin. Emma Stone uses something between a mask and sophisticated products: she moisturizes her skin with natural grape seed oil. She assured the public its effects can be more potent than those of a cream made up of over a dozen ingredients. Emmy Rossum is convinced nothing can compare to her 'skin potion': cold pressed olive oil. She spreads it on her whole body after bathing and she routinely uses it as a moisturizer for her facial skin, too. She insists that it is a substance that works wonders.

A valuable Hollywood beauty secret has 'leaked' from the famous skin expert Vera Kantor who owns the Verabella Skin Therapy Spa and has treated many celebrities such as Diane Lane, Linsday Lohan or Vanessa Hudgens. She made public her incredibly appreciated skin lifting 'trick' which consists of a double mask made up of pretty simple ingredients you can easily find anywhere. This beauty idea of hers has already been used by many Hollywood personalities, so why wouldn't you try it as well? All you need is honey (1/8 teaspoon), olive oil (a few drops), one egg (separate the yolk from the egg white), and some lemon juice (1/2 table spoon). Mix the egg yolk with all the other ingredients and apply on your clean and dry face. Keep the mask for about 10 minutes. It is extraordinarily nourishing and moisturizing. Besides, it helps you exfoliate skin. After you wash it off, you have to take the second step in your skin 'recipe'. Mix the egg white with the lemon juice this time and keep the mask for about 5 minutes. After you wash it off and clean your skin, apply your favorite serum and moisturizing cream. The second mask will tighten and brighten your skin, so it is important that you nourish your face thoroughly after you washed it off.

4. Anti-Cellulite Tips

What about skin care that combats cellulite? Strange as it may seem with so many expensive products available, some Hollywood personalities still maintain a few 'home-made' tricks. As you can picture, it is an act of courage for a Hollywood start to openly admit she has to struggle against the same problems as a 'common' woman. Take their word for granted! No celebrity would afford publicly talking about such a sensitive issue without disclosing highly effective tips.

For instance, Halle Berry confessed that she also uses her own 'recipe' for body skin: ground coffee, which increases blood flow, makes the skin smoother, and has exfoliating properties. Gwyneth Paltrow has discovered that an organic diet (devoid of any junk food) can be more valuable than expensive anti-cellulite products. She eats as natural as possible and she totally avoids fats and sweets in order to maintain a good quality of her skin. Together with regular exercise, this diet works magic on her skin. Another great suggestion for getting rid of cellulite comes from Raquel Castaneda, the celebrity make-up artist. She mentioned Rodial's Tummy Tuck Sticks, a dietary supplement that helps you speed digestion. If you take it while you also make sure you eat as healthy as possible, your waist line will be skinnier and you will definitely look better.

5. Anti-Aging Solutions

How about anti-aging secrets that keep Hollywood celebrities looking youthful and bright even after 40? Keeping your skin young and radiant is a vital aspect of skin care and several personalities have shared their routines. Take advantage of them, too! For instance, Courtney Cox's skin still looks amazing, even though she's about 50. The star uses a cream called Kinerase C8 Peptide Intensive Treatment, a potent solution against aging. This product diminishes wrinkles, brightens the skin, all stimulates cell regeneration. However this may be an anti-aging solution that you probably afford only from time to time (since one bottle costs about 100 USD), so for those of us who don't lead the life of a star, the celebrity in question also offered a second tip: Estée Laudier Time Zone line and wrinkle reducing cream. Keep it in mind as a more affordable cream that is quite well-known for its amazing rejuvenating qualities.

Sharon Stone is not only a sex symbol, but also a woman whose extremely young-looking skin and face makes you wonder what skin care methods she uses for that purpose. The actress has quite high standards in many aspects and keeping her skin young for as long as possible was one of her major goals. Dior Capture Totale is a product she shared with the public for its amazing qualities. This cream is based on a rare revitalizing plant and it can visibly reduce wrinkles, age spots, and lack of skin firmness. However it is not cheap and as an alternative you may want to consider something else: Miracle of Aloe Age Spot Fade Cream. This second product is also part of Sharon Stone's toolkit for skin care. And you must admit that she still looks incredibly young even though she's almost 60 years old.

Christie Brinkley found that make-up can also maintain skin youth both through covering up smooth lines and by means of a series of ingredients that rejuvenate the skin. Thus she recommends a product belonging to the cosmetic line Clinique. The Repair wear Anti-aging Make-up is a good idea for minimizing wrinkles. Another option she suggests for skin care is the Advances Radiance targeted at women over 30. Keep in mind such products can work on a night out when you have to conceal your ageing signs , but they are also good for keeping your skin youthful-looking for a longer time. Goldie Hawn is not really young anymore if we only judge by her biological age. And yet she still looks gorgeous for a woman belonging to her generation. What is her secret? According to what she shared with the media, her anti-aging routines rely mainly on a special oil that intensively nourishes the skin. She highly recommends a product called Dremu Oil whose skin regeneration effects are unbeatable. She is convinced it can reduce wrinkles for most women who try it, since it has proven to be such a great treatment for her skin. For those of you who are on a really tight budget, there is an alternative solution in order to avoid doing nothing for your skin: try the simple Vitamin E whose effects can be a bit similar to those of the product recommended by Goldie Hawn.

Another tip to erase some years off your face comes from the beautiful Ashley Judd who uses the cream produced by the line American Beauty (Boost Overnight Radiance Cream). This product is not very expensive and certainly you don't have to live in Hollywood to be able to purchase it. It acts upon your skin at night and it's quite effective for hydration and firming effects. If you have a few more bugs to spend, you could also try Bobbi Brown's hydrating night cream, another secret that Ashley Judd has generously made public. Can you say her face doesn't look healthy, young, and shining? Hardly.

Christina Applegate is about 40 years old and yet she looks 10 years younger, don't you think so? What are her beauty secrets? Well, she has confessed she's been using a wonderful facial cream for over 15 years, namely Crème de la Mer. She openly attributed the beauty of her skin to this unique cream created according to a concept of a NASA scientist. Its ingredients are quite special and you could not easily find a product to replace its sophisticated formula. It's based primarily on sea kelp, vitamins, and minerals combined in such an elaborate way, that it makes your skin glow and look very young. A solution that may be slightly more affordable however is Olay Regenerist Deep Hydration Cream, another product recommended by Christina Applegate. This cream has similar hydrating properties and, in case the product mentioned earlier is too much of a dream for you, it's quite wise to use this one instead.

Sarah Jessica Parker considers Lancôme to be exceptional cosmetic line that she advises us to try out on our own skin. Her favorite anti-aging solution is Rénergie Microlift Eye R.A.R.E, a cream with awesome lifting properties. Catherine Zeta-Jones has two basic solutions to stay young. Her first tip is a cream produced by the Elizabeth Arden line – Prevage Anti-ageing Treatment. However it costs over 100 USD, so you may want to buy it rarely as a luxury product only. To make up for this extremely good, but Hollywood-priced idea with a second tip, Catherine Zeta-Jones also mentioned the line Neutrogena. The cream she uses is called Ageless Restauratives Age Reverse Night Cream and she is quite proud of its effects on her skin.

Halle Berry has a few skin care tips that she uses even though still quite young. Her routines center on skin toning and exfoliating. For this purpose she uses a fruit acid solution twice a day immediately after washing her skin, then she nourishes her skin with a rich moisturizer. Her preferred product is Burt's Bees Radiance Daily Cleanser which doesn't cost too much and could be purchased by everyone. Murad AHA/BHA Exfoliating Cleanser is a more expensive option for a similar routine, should you have a larger budget for your skin care. Both products are fully recommended by Halle Berry who is quite satisfied with the way such a solution increases skin radiance and promotes normal cell turnover.

6. Hollywood Hair Care

When it comes to hair care, many of us are probably tempted to think Hollywood beauty is mainly about applying intensive hair dye as often as possible, changing colors and looks, and visiting one's personal stylist as often as possible. Nevertheless that's not what celebrities say when they are asked about what keeps their hair so healthy and so wonderfully looking. The truth is hair care is just as complex as skin care and there is much to learn from Hollywood personalities if we want to equal their beauty in a natural way.

Let's start with a few suggestions that account for the beauty of Natalie Portman's hair: a silicone-based serum should be mixed with a good hair conditioner in order to leave your hair shiny and healthy. Another celebrity who uses this hair care formula is January Jones. It is considered to be a powerful tip to enhance the effects of a normal conditioner with strong shine and smoothness. This mixture should stay on your hair for about 15 minutes after you have just washed it. Rinse out thoroughly and enjoy your hair afterwards! This tip should be practiced at least every other week if you want to have gorgeous hair.

A favorite of many celebrities is the **John Masters Organics** cosmetic line. While some personalities also enjoy skin care products, quite a few have mentioned this line when asked about what they use to keep their hair healthy. For instance, Thandie Newton said she loves the Lavander and Avocado intensive Conditioner. In this product organic oil from the two basic plants are combined with other 10 extracts from natural products to create an extremely nourishing balm for dry or damaged hair. The actress also uses the Citrus and Neroli detangler which can be used as a leave-in or as a rinse-out conditioner. It is based on numerous organic extracts such as soy protein, borage oil, and grapefruit, lemon, and neroli extracts which will charm you with their aroma.

Oliver Thornton mentioned the Lavander and Rosemary shampoo as a major part of his hair care routine. Produced by the same cosmetic organic line, this shampoo is wonderful as a basis for keeping healthy hair. It combines 13 certified organic ingredients and it is optimal for normal hair. It does not contain sodium lauryl sulfate and it is extremely smooth and soothing for your hair. It makes your hair shiny and strong. Georgina Chapman prefers the Evening Primrose Shampoo for dry hair. Not only does it contain numerous plant extracts, but also it uses organic oil to nourish and moisturize your hair while preventing damage. It is also amazing for colored hair, as it has a powerful healing effect on the scalp as well as the hair itself.

If there's any fact on which most celebrities agree is that you have to use natural masks for your hair so as to keep it healthy. It's not enough to treat your hair with conditioner and shampoo, no matter how good the products you use are. A method that works just as well is lubricating it with organic nourishing oil (e.g. olive oil or coconut oil). All you have to do is place 1-3- tablespoons oil in a bowl and then spread it through your whole hair with your fingers. Cover your head with a towel and let the organic oil spread into your hair and feed it from its tips to its root all night long. Gently wash and condition your hair the next morning.

Argan oil is an extremely powerful weapon in the toolkit of many Hollywood celebrities. Numerous Hollywood stylists recommend it together with personalities who turned it into one if their most magic secrets. It has great nourishing properties and it can give back shine and health even to badly damaged hair. In case you have used too many chemically-laden hair-dyeing products, organic argan oil is certainly your cure. For example, Marian Cottilard loves the Sultan de Saba Argan Oil which contains 99% organic oil along with rose and vitamin E. Many top celebrities use the argan oil for their skin, too. It is quite lightweight and it doesn't charge the skin with too many fatty acids. Instead it soothes and moisturizes it. Argan oil is the ideal organic product for both skin care and hair care and Hollywood cosmeticians and stars are quite familiar with its power. For instance, a hair care brand such as Morrocanoil relies heavily on this substance for intensive hair care. It's about time you started benefiting from its gifts, too!

One way to use it in a pleasant fashion is pouring a few drops of oil into your usual conditioner and thus let it subtly nourish your hair every two days or so. Ideally you could also us3e this amazing balm for your hair every day. However there are some people whose hair has oily tendencies and a less frequent use may be advisable. The best method is to let the oil spread into your hair for almost half an hour. For this reason it is also important to use a quality conditioner, because all its ingredients will penetrate your hair together with the nourishing argan oil. For people who have normal to dry hair a bona fide treatment with this amazing argan oil can also take the form of a hair mask to leave in overnight. Gently massage a few table spoons of argan oil into your hair, pressing softly with your fingertips at the root in order to let the oil have a thorough effect. Cover your head with a large towel and wash your hair the next morning. Your hair will look wonderfully shiny and silky.

Kareena Kapoor has shared with us her secret hair care routine. Apart from the famous **Kerastase** shampoo (which is also recommended by other celebs such as Kristin Stewart), this personality has her own hair mask which guarantees long-term health and beauty for her hair. She oils her hair once a month with a combination of castor, coconut, and almond oil. If you think your hair is too dry, you can experiment with this potent blend even more often. Try it out and you'll notice the effect by yourself! Another valuable product from the same beauty line is the Kerastase Masque Oleo Relax which can be used once a week for treating dry and damaged hair.

A hair care line which is extremely appreciated by Hollywood celebrities is **Kiehl**. You can start with the Olive Fruit Oil Deeply Repairation Hair Pack for a holistic take on hair care, especially if your hair is damaged or dull. The Kiehl leave-in Hair Conditioner is also remarkably good. As for split end treatment, many celebrities prefer using Loreal Paris Everstrong Overnight Repair Treatment. For a more strongly organic solution, you can try the Macadamia Natural Oil Deep Repair Mask. Your hair will become very soft and silky after using this product.

7. Detox Weight Loss Programs

Organic Juice may sound like too much of a simple element to include in your diet when you want to lose weight but you can take its powers for granted! Many Hollywood personalities such as Zooey Dechanel or Gwen Stephani resort to pressed juice in order to stay fit. Of course if you need to get rid of 5 kg in 4-6 days, you may want to consider some harsher diets based on high calorie restrictions. However as a maintenance tip, pressed juiced has proved to be very useful. All you have to do is drink six juices per day for several weeks in a row (or how long you want). Ideally you should drink your juice between meals and of course don't eat fatty products, junk food, or sweets. Stay as natural as you can. Actually pressed juice will make sure some of your usual hunger is satiated

If you want to lose weight fast, you can try drinking exclusively pressed juice. It is possible and it does wonders! Just keep in mind your body should be very healthy and 'saturated' with minerals and vitamins before you start your pressed juice cleanse. Your immunity should be high and you should avoid going on such a diet during periods of high stress (e.g. exams, job changes etc.). This weight loss and energy boosting secret is recommended by great Hollywood names such as Salma Hayek, Nicole Richie, and Gwyneth Paltrow who, as you can well see, look totally amazing. How could you not try this diet, at least to see what effects it has on your own body? You can use any fruit and vegetables, just make sure you diversify your detox diet. You should not limit yourself only to products with a high Vitamin C content, for instance. Try strawberries, banana, cucumber, tomato, kiwi etc. during the same day.

The So-Cal cleanse has many fans among Hollywood celebrities. Denise Richards, Jessica Simpson, Michelle Williams are just a few names of personalities who have testified that this detox program is highly recommendable. This cleanse includes a plan for 30 days that implies the elimination of meat, dairy products, white flour, caffeine, and alcohol. Instead it focuses on a series of supplements that will help you lose weight while maintaining your body in a state of good health. This plan is not the easiest solution in terms of cost, since you'll have to purchase the supplements and that will mean getting rid of about 400 USD for one whole package. However keep it in mind as a detox program that has proven effective and that is widely appreciated and practiced by celebrities such as Channing Tatum or Mila Kunis who have openly praised it. Cynthia Pasquella, the certified nutritionist who invented this famous cleanse, has already explained why she decided to make her program so long (and a month does seem quite a long time to go without meat or dairy). In her opinion one week is not enough for a real detox – it is a rather artificial method of cleansing the body. For this reason she prefers a slower and longer plan that acts upon the body and its metabolism in depth. Pasquella also claimed that juice cleanses only operate on the body in a superficial level, as their cleansing effects only help it release toxins. In her opinion you shouldn't stop there, but get to the second and third phase of cleansing so as to eliminate all the toxins, even those that are stored in fat cells. Although there are many celebrities who advocate the So-Cal cleanse, it is recommendable that you only practice it if you are thoroughly healthy, because living for one whole month without any meat and dairy may be a bit problematic. It is optimal to consult a specialist before starting the detox. If you get the confirmation that there's no risk to your body to follow this deep cleansing program, you can rest assured you will also lose considerable weight after you complete the 30-day program.

Gwyneth Paltrow is an ardent supporter of the detox diet. Her personal preference that she completely incorporated in her lifestyle is Alejandro Junger's Clean program, a 21-day diet that is oriented more towards cleansing the body and keeping it healthy rather than weight loss. Nevertheless one of the invaluable 'side effects' of this program is that you will also get rid of a few kilos if you practice it. Actually provided that you follow all its rules, you will easily lose undesired weight and, more importantly, you will stay fit. This program consists of one main meal (lunch) for which you have to choose a few products from a given list of permitted food. The rest of your day will only include one shake in the morning and another in the evening. Its main advantage is an extraordinarily powerful cleansing effect of your whole body and a good regulation of your metabolism.

Beyonce and Jay Z have adopted a vegan detox program that spreads on 22 days. Beyonce has a body to die for and yet she is not naturally very thin, as you can notice yourself. She has to strive to stay slim and fit. Despite her body type (extremely attractive without any doubt), Beyonce managed to lose 20 pounds in less than 2 weeks for her role in the movie *Dreamgirls*. How did she do that? Well, she used precisely her now famous vegan detox diet. Her diet is based on a Master Cleanse that consists only of hot water, lemon juice, maple syrup, and cayenne pepper for 10 days. It is definitely not easy to follow, but such a detox diet is incredibly effective and powerful. The bottom line is that, if you succeed in going on such a diet for 10 days, repeating this process a bit later is going to prove quite easy. It is the first steps that seem difficult, since your brain is not yet used to the idea of letting your body live only on this Master Cleanse.

A variation of the Master Cleanse is the LemonAid, a concentrate created by David Kirsch, a famous nutritionist and personal trainer of many Hollywood celebrities. The neat advantage of this invention is that it offers you your daily product as such and you save a lot of time. You get a concentrate of lemon, maple syrup, and cayenne pepper already prepared. Anne Hathaway practices this diet on a shorter term. She uses Dr. Kirsch's plan as a 48-hour detox before she has to get on the red carpet. All she has to do is ingest this ready-made concentrate 4 times a day without eating anything.

8. Top Celebrity Diet Secrets

If you are looking for some more easy and 'tolerant' weight loss tips and you don't want to put too much pressure on your body, you can simply include a few tips in your daily routines. It's true that you will get rid of unwanted kilos more slowly, but, according to what many celebrities say, the effect is quite sure.

For instance, you can drink plenty of water. Elle McPherson drinks one liter of water each morning, right after she gets out of bed. Do you think she is called 'The Body' for no reason? Gwyneth Paltrow and Cate Blanchet are also admirers of this beauty trick that is recommended by Dr. Nish Joshi, a famous British nutritionist. Ideally you should drink 2 liters of water every day.

Another great weapon against weight is green tea, as you probably already know. There's no limit to green tea: drink as much as you want, but make sure it is at least 2 liters every day. You should purchase some quality authentic green tea from reliable stores. Dita von Teese has adopted this drink as part of her daily routine. She drinks a cup of green tea every morning. However famous nutritionists such as Rachel Beller and Mark Stephens recommend drinking even a higher quantity for its amazing anti-oxidant, energizing, and cleansing effects. In their opinion one should drink about 8 cups/glasses of green tea every day, if one really wants to get rid of surplus weight. In order to make your experience more pleasant, you can use different types of green tea in combinations with orange blossom, lemon, ginger, ginseng, cherry blossom etc. All these natural substances will only add to the powerful and unbeatable effect of green tea and you will not get bored of its taste after you integrate this drink in your routine.

You can also replace green tea with another Hollywood weight loss secret, namely oolong tea. Personalities such as Oprah and Rachel Ray can testify it works extremely well for weight loss. It contains a high amount of anti-oxidants that will boost your metabolism. Your body will burn fat much faster than usual, especially in your tummy and upper arm areas. Scientists have discovered that, once you reach your ideal weight, drinking oolong tea on a regular basis as part of your daily routine will help you maintain your desired weight. Its substances will block the fat-building enzymes in your body. Moreover, oolong tea has a high concentration of caffeine and you can use it to energize your brain instead of coffee in the morning or after lunch. It's sugar-free, it tastes great, and it is also calorie-free – the perfect substitute for coffee!

Hollywood celebrities such Kate Perry, Lady Gaga, Eva Mendez, and Megan Fox prefer the 5-factor Diet when they want to lose weight. It was designed by the celebrity trainer Harley Pasternak and it has spread very fast worldwide as a highly efficient weight loss tip. It is based on the idea that in order to lose weight, you have to eat 5 meals per day with recipes containing maximum 5 ingredients. All the meals must include 5 elements: protein, fiber, complex carbs, fat, and fluids.

Kim Kardashian confessed her trick is the Atkins diet, while also admitting she has sometimes allowed herself to 'cheat' and include a forbidden food in her initial plan. After she had her baby the celebrity had to lose weight fast in order to look her best again. The Atkins diet is based on the golden rule of cutting out carbs and eating lots of protein instead. If you follow this rule, calories won't be so much of a problem. This diet has worked for many people, but of course it is also advisable to reduce your food intake. You don't have to count calories and starve; however you do have to show a lot of moderation in your eating habits, if you really want this diet to work. Eating 5-6 stuffed meals per day may not result in the desired weight loss.

9. Conclusion

This book is a tool for staying Hollywood healthy by guiding yourself according to several tips that famous celebrities have made public. While you will probably not be able to adopt all the secrets that we shared with you in this book, given your quite different lifestyle, Hollywood is definitely a great pool of resources for beauty and weight loss. You should start with the tips that meet your highest demands and necessities. Are you perhaps a bit overweight? Do you fear the effects of the ageing process? Does your hair look dry and damaged because you dye it quite often? Have you tried many chemically-laden cosmetic products, from your day cream to lifting serums and have grown quite tired of promises that don't come true? Do you feel you are paying too much for products that may not be worth their price?

It's quite understandable if you have been a bit confused about the best cosmetic solutions for your facial skin, your hair, or your body. We live in a world in which we are bombarded with myriad products and publicity doesn't often help us too much. We may be distrustful of its devices and we may want to invest our money wisely instead of wasting it by eternally experimenting till we find the best solution. This book was meant to help you precisely in this effort to find the optimal methods to stay healthy. By looking into the organic products that Hollywood celebrities have declared exceptionally efficient, you have a guarantee of quality. Your next step is actually starting your personal beauty routines in concordance with Hollywood tips. Get Hollywood healthy and beautiful and make sure you share your own secrets afterwards, so that others can also benefit from them as well!

Thank You so much for reading this book, if it gave you a ton of value it would be amazing for you to leave a REVIEW!

CLICK THIS LINK TO CLAIM YOUR 100% FREE GIFT !